Table of Contents

Introduction

Herpes simplex is a virus. That means that there isn't a known "cure" that will prevent symptoms from returning. But there are things you can do to find relief during an HSV-1 or HSV-2 outbreak.You may be able to reduce inflammation, irritation, and other symptoms through a mix of lifestyle changes and dietary supplements.However, these remedies aren't a replacement for a clinical treatment plan.

Herpes Simplex

The herpes simplex virus, also known as HSV, is an infection that causes herpes. Herpes can appear in various parts of the body, most commonly on the genitals or mouth. There are two types of the herpes simplex virus.

• HSV-1: primarily causes oral herpes, and is generally responsible for cold sores and fever blisters around the mouth and on the face.

• HSV-2: primarily causes genital herpes, and is generally responsible for genital herpes outbreaks.

The herpes simplex virus is a contagious virus that can be transmitted from person to person through direct contact. Children will often contract HSV-1 from early contact with an infected adult. They then carry the virus with them for the rest of their lives.

HSV-1

HSV-1 can be contracted from general interactions such as:

• eating from the same utensils

• sharing lip balm

• kissing

The virus spreads more quickly when an infected person is experiencing an outbreak. An estimated 67 percent of people ages 49 or younger are seropositive for HSV-1, though they may never experience an outbreak. It's also possible to get genital herpes from HSV-1 if someone who performed oral sex had cold sores during that time.

HSV-2

HSV-2 is contracted through forms of sexual contact with a person who has HSV-2. An estimated 20 percent of sexually active adults in the United States are infected with HSV-2, according to the American Academy of Dermatology (AAD). HSV-2 infections are spread through contact with a herpes sore. In contrast, most people get HSV-1 from an infected person who is asymptomatic, or does not have sores.

Risk Of Developing Herpes Simplex Infections

Anyone can be infected with HSV, regardless of age. Your risk is based almost entirely on exposure to the infection. In cases of sexually transmitted HSV, people are more at risk when they have sex not protected by condoms or other barrier methods. Other risk factors for HSV-2 include:

• having multiple sex partners

• having sex at a younger age

• being female

• having another sexually transmitted infection (STI)

• having a weakened immune system

If a pregnant woman is having an outbreak of genital herpes at the time of childbirth, it can expose the baby to both types of HSV, and may put them at risk for serious complications.

Recognizing The Signs Of Herpes Simplex

It's important to understand that someone may not have visible sores or symptoms and still be infected by the virus. They may also transmit the virus to others. Some of the symptoms associated with this virus include:

• blistering sores (in the mouth or on the genitals)

• pain during urination (genital herpes)

• itching

You may also experience symptoms that are similar to the flu. These symptoms can include:

• fever

• swollen lymph nodes

• headaches

• tiredness

• lack of appetite

HSV can also spread to the eyes, causing a condition called herpes keratitis. This can cause symptoms such as eye pain, discharge, and a gritty feeling in the eye.

Herpes Simplex Diagnosis

This type of virus is generally diagnosed with a physical exam. Your doctor may check your body for sores and ask you about some of your symptoms. Your doctor may also request HSV testing. This is known as a herpes culture. It will confirm the diagnosis if you have sores on your genitals. During this test, your doctor will take a swab sample of fluid from the sore and then send it to a laboratory for testing. Blood tests for antibodies to HSV-1 and HSV-2 can also help diagnose these infections. This is especially helpful when there are no sores present.

Herpes Simplex Treatment

There is currently no cure for this virus. Treatment focuses on getting rid of sores and limiting outbreaks. It's possible that your sores will go away without treatment. However, your doctor may determine you need one or more of the following medications:

• acyclovir

• famciclovir

• valacyclovir

These medications can help people infected with the virus reduce the risk of transmitting it to others. The medications also help to lower the intensity and frequency of outbreaks. These medications may come in oral (pill) form, or may be applied as a cream. For severe outbreaks, these medications may also be administered by injection.

Long-Term Outlook For Herpes Simplex

People who become infected with HSV will have the virus for the rest of their lives. Even if it does not manifest symptoms, the virus will continue to live in an infected person's nerve cells. Some people may experience regular outbreaks. Others will only experience one outbreak after they have been infected and then the virus may become dormant. Even if a virus is dormant, certain stimuli can trigger an outbreak. These include:

• stress

• menstrual periods

• fever or illness

• sun exposure or sunburn

It's believed that outbreaks may become less intense over time because the body starts creating antibodies. If a generally healthy person is infected with the virus, there are usually no complications.

Preventing The Spread Of Herpes Simplex Infections

Although there is no cure for herpes, you can take measures to avoid contracting the virus, or to prevent transmitting HSV to another person. If you're experiencing an outbreak of HSV-1, consider taking a few preventive steps:

• Try to avoid direct physical contact with other people.

• Don't share any items that can pass the virus around, such as cups, towels, silverware, clothing, makeup, or lip balm.

• Don't participate in oral sex, kissing, or any other type of sexual activity during an outbreak.

• Wash your hands thoroughly and apply medication with cotton swabs to reduce contact with sores.

People with HSV-2 should avoid any type of sexual activity with other people during an outbreak. If the person is not experiencing symptoms but has been diagnosed with the virus, a condom should be used during intercourse. But even when using a condom, the virus can still be passed to a partner from uncovered skin. Women who are pregnant and infected may have to take medication to prevent the virus from infecting their unborn babies.

Natural Remedy

Natural Herpes Treatment Option

Alright, it's time to get rid of this nasty little bugger once and for all. So, here's the strongest natural herpes cure you'll come across, along with the all-important scientific validation on why it works so amazingly well. Pharmaceutical company confirms… "Olive Leaf Extract Killed Every Virus, Bacteria and Protozoa They Tested it Against!" Back in 1969, Dr Harold Renis was working for the Upjohn Company (now owned by Pfizer) and was doing a lot of research into the therapeutic benefits of olive leaf extract (OLE). Once this pharmaceutical company realized the astonishing health benefits of olive leaf extract, they tried to obtain a patent on it and claim it as a drug. Of course, they were unsuccessful (how can you get a patent on a natural substance). So once this happened, they stopped all research into OLE and quickly poo-pooed it. Unfortunately for them, they'd already let the cat out of the bag and supplement companies began to jump on the olive leaf extract band wagon and started producing it in supplemental form. The main substance in OLE is Oleuropein and this is what destroys the virus. It basically puts a force field around the virus and infected cells so they cannot continue to grow and replicate. Here's the 3 main benefits of using olive leaf extract for herpes as quoted by the Olivus website…

• Has the ability to interfere with critical amino acid production essential for viruses. Shown to kill oral and genital herpes virus and herpes zoster virus (shingles/chicken pox).

• Has the ability to contain viral infection and/or spread by inactivating viruses or by preventing virus shedding, budding, or assembly at the cell membrane.

• Ability to directly penetrate infected cells and stop the symptoms of herpes by shutting down viral replication in male & female herpes and mild herpes simplex, zoster, type 1 and type 2.

The French Also Discovered the Remarkable Benefits of Olive Leaf Extract as a Treatment for Herpes

In 1992, French biologists "found that all of the herpes viruses were inhibited, killed, or cured by extracts from olive leaf". Their findings were also backed up by the citing of 28 references on the anti-viral qualities of Oleuropein in their report. So this was not some willy-nilly study. It was very precise and very detailed (and they actually used both the "killed" and "cure" words in this report). Along with shutting down and killing viruses, including the herpes simplex virus, the other powerful benefit of olive leaf extract is it boosts the immune system tremendously. In fact, you would be hard pressed to find anything out there that works better. This is another reason why OLE will protect you from virtually every ailment that exists, including the common cold and flu virus. Even Aids sufferers are finding incredible relief from the use of olive leaf extract. It really is the "cure-all compound of the 21st century!"

Olive leaf advocate, Dr. James Privitera, has given OLE to many of his patients infected with the herpes simplex virus and seen some remarkable results. One of his male patients experienced frequent lesions, along with constant fatigue for many years after becoming infected. But within a week of taking OLE his lesions disappeared and his energy levels increased dramatically. He even wrote to Dr. Privitera to say that olive leaf was the only medicine that eliminated his herpes. He stated... "Even the most minute blisters are totally gone!". And in a 1993 private herpes study of six participants, all reported symptomatic relief and three of the subjects said their lesions were completely gone within 48 hours from treatment with olive leaf extract. The icing on the cake was all six participants said this option produced far better results than medications they have previously used such as Acyclovir, Zorvirax, and Valtrex.

How Much Olive Leaf Extract Do You Need to Take and for How Long?

As a herpes treatment, you need to know just how much OLE to take for it to be effective and for how long. First off, the dosage for olive leaf extract will depend on the potency of the product you buy. OLE comes in a variety of potencies, from "regular" to "super strength". We advise you stay well clear of the regular potencies as they are often too weak and will not destroy the herpes simplex virus. Instead, go for the super strength varieties that have a pure Oleuropein extract content of 25% or more (250 mg's of pure oleuropein). If they contain added dry olive leaf powder for extra strength then even better. For this reason, we recommend Olivus OLE to all of our clients. It's by far the strongest and most absorbable olive leaf extract you'll find anywhere in the world - and it works incredibly well on the herpes simplex virus! You can view their website here for more information.

Note: Because the super strength Olivus OLE (OliveLeafMax) capsules work so well, demand is extremely high for this product, and unfortunately, they regularly sell out. If you find this is the case then you can go on their waiting list. You will need to be patient, but it's well worth it!

Update: Due to Olivus regularly running out of their high strength olive leaf extract, we have been forced to look for an alternative product that is as good (if not better) as what they are supplying. This brand is definitely it... Real European OLE Super Strength 25% Oleuropean. This olive leaf extract is extremely high quality and very high potency. You cannot go wrong taking either the Olivus or Real European OLE.

How to Consume Olive Leaf Extract

Now, when it comes to how much OLE to take you need to keep in mind that olive leaf extract is not harmful, even at high dosages. It's considered safe to use so don't be afraid of "overdosing". In this case you actually need to be more concerned with "underdosing!" So we suggest you take at least the highest recommended daily amount suggested on the bottle (on an empty stomach) for the first 6-9 months, then as your symptoms disappear, drop back to the suggested maintenance dose after that. You will definitely need to hit the virus hard to destroy it and this approach is the most effective way to accomplish this. For the Olivus

OliveLeafMax capsules, the recommended dose for eliminating viruses is 4-6 capsules per day taken in divided amounts. For the Real European brand, it's 3-4 capsules daily.

Watch Out for Herxheimers Reaction

It should be noted here that for some people, olive leaf extract can make them feel queasy and even cause mild diarrhea. Because OLE is such a powerful detoxifier, if you have a high viral load or a lot of pathogens in your body, you can experience something called herxheimers reaction. This is simply a "die-off" reaction that occurs and is basically the body's immune response to the release of toxins caused by the eradication of these harmful pathogens. Herxheimers reaction resembles "flu-like" symptoms and usually lasts for around 5-7 days. But this short-lived side effect is actually a sign that the treatment is working (which is a good thing of course) so don't be discouraged by it. Instead, drink plenty of water to help flush the toxins out of the body because once this "detox" is over, we guarantee you'll start to feel better than you've felt in a long time! So, if herxheimers reaction does happen to you and it does hit you hard, we suggest you drop back to the lowest dose recommended on the bottle and then slowly build the dosage back up over a 2-3-week period to the highest recommended daily amount. You then stay on the highest amount for a further 6-9 months to ensure a thorough cleanse. Once this period is over, you will then continue on the maintenance dose (suggested maintenance dose on the bottle) indefinitely. And what exactly do we mean by "indefinitely"? Yes, we mean for the rest of your life! Even though OLE will kill the herpes virus, we still suggest you continue to take it every day for what we like to call "health insurance". This is not actually a "prescription" we're talking about here anyway; this is a treatment that's designed to not only cure your herpes for good, but also boost your overall health and wellness and help you live a longer life. So, remember this... The powerful benefits of olive leaf extract go way beyond just treating and curing the herpes virus. Please take the time to read this important article on the benefits of OLE and its amazing curative powers... Olive Leaf Extract - The Remedy of Choice for Thousands of Years.

Final Note: Olive leaf extract is also an excellent topical treatment for herpes blisters. You can buy it in tincture form or powdered form (mix with a slight amount of oregano oil) and use this to rub directly on any sores or blisters for some extra fast healing and relief!

Other Permanent Treatment Options For Herpes

There are other natural remedies for herpes that work exceptionally well. We suggest you use these in conjunction with your olive leaf extract to totally destroy this unwelcome parasite for good…

Natural Herpes Cure: Colloidal Silver

Colloidal silver works in a similar way to olive leaf extract. The positively charged ions in colloidal silver bind to the protein structure surrounding the virus so it can't replicate. In addition, if the particles contained in the colloidal silver are small enough (less than 6 nanometers), they will penetrate the virus and attach themselves to the genetic material contained within it. This also stops the herpes virus from being able to replicate even further and basically "starves" it. So by doing this, the viral infection is quickly contained and quarantined. The truth is, by combining colloidal silver with olive leaf extract, oregano oil and BHT (see next two cures), you actually have the most powerful herpes destroyer combo that exists on this planet! In fact, you'll be hard pressed to find a more potent and astonishingly effective treatment for eradicating the herpes virus anywhere. We guarantee it! According to Homeopath and colloidal silver expert, Dr Robert Scott Bell, to get your daily dose of colloidal silver, you must take a supplement that contains silver in a form of at least 10 parts per million (particles at 6 nanometers or less). We know of only one colloidal silver brand on the market that not only fits this criterion, but actually goes way further to deliver the most potent colloidal silver supplement you'll ever come across (particles at 0.8 nanometers). It's called Sovereign Silver. One reviewer on the Earth Clinic website had this to say about Sovereign Silver for eradicating herpes... "I found out that colloidal silver kills all viruses, bacteria and fungus - I had herpes and took a teaspoon of colloidal silver (sovereign silver) 5 times a day for 3 months and it is gone. I found out that the brand of silver is very important. I have been re-checked and I am negative for herpes. I was amazed to find that this disease can be cured." For dosages, take one teaspoon (5 ml's) of colloidal silver (hold under tongue for 30 seconds then swallow) 5 times a day for 3 months. After this, take one teaspoon twice daily for a further 9 months. Also remember to never use a metal teaspoon when measuring out your dosage as the metals in the spoon react negatively with the silver particles. Use a BPA free plastic spoon or measuring cup instead. In addition to taking the colloidal silver orally, you can also apply colloidal silver topically on any lesions for quicker healing and relief.

Natural Herpes Treatment Option: Oregano Oil

Oregano oil is a strong antiviral and antibacterial substance that has been proven to kill the herpes virus in test tube studies. This oil (the 100% pure oil) contains two powerful compounds, carvacrol and thymol, and these are the essential ingredients that destroy the virus. Carvacrol is especially important and the higher the levels of this compound the better. Like we said, when combined with olive leaf extract, colloidal silver and BHT, oregano oil is unbeatable. But and this is crucial, you must make sure you purchase the right type of oregano oil and use it correctly (drops under the tongue, added to water and applied to the base of the spine). This is extremely important as you will not benefit from it unless you do! The oregano oil MUST be the "super strength" 100% pure Mediterranean oil.Nothing else will work.This oregano oil is very reasonably priced and actually contains some of the highest levels of carvacol and thymol we've come across so far (up to 92% carvacrol!). To use the oregano oil correctly and get the most out of it, here's what you need to do (be sure to follow this plan exactly). Firstly, mix up a small batch of oregano oil and virgin coconut oil to apply externally to the base of the spine. You can also add a small amount of DMSO to this mix as well.As far as an exact ratio? Only you can work this out. If you use too much coconut oil it won't be strong enough, however, if you don't use enough the oregano oil may burn. The mix should be strong enough so you feel a tingling sensation but not a burning sensation. 3-4 drops of oregano oil added to a teaspoon of coconut oil is a rough ballpark figure. Once you have your mix, apply this to the bottom portion of the spine, from the tailbone to the top of the buttocks area (roughly 2-3-inch area). Rub on gently and leave on for as long as possible. Secondly, add 4-5 drops of oregano oil to a minimum 8 oz glass of clean filtered water and drink down. The more water the less it will burn and the better it will taste. Do this twice daily on an empty stomach. Thirdly, mix in 2-3 drops of oregano oil in roughly one teaspoon of virgin coconut oil. Take this and hold under the tongue for 10-15 minutes. Make sure you dilute the oregano oil enough with coconut oil or it may burn the bottom of your mouth. Once again, you should only feel a slight tingling, not a burning sensation. Be sure to do this at least once a day. Finally, take one day off per week from the oregano oil to give your body a chance to recuperate. The oregano oil is a powerful detoxifier so taking a break once a week will allow the body to rest and recharge.

Natural Herpes Cure: BHT (Butylated Hydroxytoluene)

Back in the mid 1980's, a scientific paper was published in the prestigious Science journal showing that a common food preservative, BHT (Butylated hydroxytoluene), could prevent lipid coated viruses from infecting their targeted cells. Since around half of all serious (viral) diseases are associated with or caused by lipid-coated viruses, this was a powerful finding. When a virus cannot invade and infect a cell, it cannot grow and replicate and will eventually die. The herpes family of viruses (along with hepatitis B & C, influenza, HIV, AIDS, and even the Ebola virus) are lipid coated viruses and all respond very well to BHT therapy. BHT is also terrific for reducing and completely stopping all herpes outbreaks. When you start detoxing the body and using powerful substances such as the olive leaf extract, colloidal silver and oregano oil, it's very common for outbreaks to occur - especially in the beginning. The virus has been lying dormant and has now been woken up. It's not happy! So, when it leaves the infected area it can, and usually does, go on a rampage at your expense. The body also begins to fight back, which further exacerbates the problem. But BHT quickly destroys the viral outbreak and produces rapid healing. In an article by researcher Ed Sharp he stated… "Inspired by early scientific reports on the antiviral activity of BHT, a number of people suffering from herpes began to experiment on themselves. As described in several books published a few years later, the BHT experimenters discovered that a daily dose of 250 to 1000 mg resulted in rapid recovery from herpes eruptions with no recurrences." Many people have used BHT to treat their herpes and then tested negative for the virus. Here's one interesting account… "Roger first began taking BHT in 1984 after reading about it in Pearson and Shaw's groundbreaking book 'Life Extension: A Practical Scientific Approach.' Initially he took about 1 gram per day because he was buying BHT in bulk at the time and larger amounts were easier to measure out than smaller ones. Later he was able to obtain BHT in capsules containing 250 mg per cap, and from that point on he took 250 mg every day for 6 to 7 years. Not surprisingly, during this period he remained completely free of herpes eruptions. More surprising is that he still remains herpes-free to this day, 19 years after his last dose of BHT. Around 6 years ago Roger had a comprehensive physical exam, including blood work. His physician told him that no antibodies to the herpes simplex virus could be found in his system."

How to Get the Most Out of BHT

So BHT supplementation is definitely another crucial link in your "herpes cure" arsenal. And the good thing about BHT is it's not expensive and is easily obtainable. There are a few precautions though and a specific way to begin taking BHT so your body can adjust to it. Firstly, you MUST combine BHT with the herb, St. John's Wort. St. John's Wort contains a substance called hypericin, and the theory (yes, it's only a theory at this stage) is that hypericin has the ability to travel down the ganglia nerve, so when it's combined with BHT it acts as a carrier to get the BHT into the area where the herpes virus likes to hide (hypericin is also a strong antidepressant too). In addition to this, because BHT is fat soluble, it should be taken with a small amount of organic virgin coconut oil (1/4 to 1/2 tablespoon) for maximum absorption, along with a daily dose of around 10,000 mg's of vitamin C. You can purchase BHT in either capsule or granule form. We recommend the capsules…. High Strength BHT Capsules. They're much easier to take and you know the exact amount you're taking each time. So begin with 250 mg's a day and stick with this amount for 3-4 days, then increase to 500 mg's per day. Once again, stay with this amount for 3-4 days before increasing to 750 mg's. After another 3-4 days increase to the maximum recommended long-term dosage of 1000 mg's per day. Stay on this for 6 months before dropping back to 500 mg's a day for another 6 months. You can then take 250 mg's of BHT every day after this period for as long as you wish. In addition to this, BHT expert, Dr Ward Dean, M.D., recommends you up the dose of BHT to 2000 mg's a day (taken in divided amounts) when experiencing a breakout to shorten the duration, so you may want to consider this recommendation if you experience a BO. The St. John's Wort must contain at least 0.3% standardized hypericin extract for it to be effective… St John's Wort 0.3% Hypericin Capsules. This supplement should be taken at a daily dose of between 900 and 1500 mg's (total for the day) in divided amounts. And of course, make sure you always take the St. John's Wort together with the BHT and coconut oil for maximum assimilation and benefit. Keep in mind that St. John's Wort is not recommended for pregnant or nursing mothers.

Note: Do not consume alcohol whilst taking BHT as BHT heightens the effects of alcohol. BHT can also thin the blood initially (if you haven't taken it before), which is why you should follow the directions and slowly build up the dose. This blood thinning is not detrimental to your health though and usually only occurs for the first 2-3 days while your body is acclimatising to it. Of course, if you're taking anticoagulant drugs, have liver problems, or blood clotting disorders such as hemophilia, you should check with your health care professional before taking BHT, just to be on the safe side.

The herpes simplex virus absolutely hates the amino acid L-Lysine. Vitamin C and zinc have also been shown to help keep the herpes virus away, along with giving the immune system a significant boost. Taking these three in supplemental form is crucial as you will need high dosages. 1000 milligrams of a high-quality lysine supplement three times a day is needed to get the virus under control, along with around 5000 milligrams of two-staged time release vitamin C and 5000 milligrams of ascorbic acid per day (yes, that's a total of 10,000 mg's of vitamin C each day!) Colloidal zinc or chelated zinc (50 mg's a day) is also recommended for optimal results. Once the virus is under control, drop down to a maintenance dose of between 500-1000 mg's per day of the lysine for 3 months before dropping it completely. Continue to eat lysine rich foods such as organic free range eggs and organic fruits and vegetables though, along with taking a wheat grass or chlorella supplement every day to raise your pH level (which also helps to kill the virus) and to remove the heavy metals from your body (which the virus likes to attach itself to). The zinc and vitamin C should be taken at the maximum dosages listed above for the full 12 months.

Natural Herpes Cure: Elderberry

Elderberry is yet another incredible remedy and treatment for herpes. This herb contains some very strong antioxidant flavonoids that are known to boost the immune system quite rapidly. It also possesses some excellent anti-viral qualities and has been shown in studies to actually stop the replication of four strains of the herpes simplex virus, including two strains that are resistant to the most common herpes pharmaceutical medication acyclovir (Zovirax).[8] In addition, elderberry is one of the best natural remedies for colds and flu you'll ever come across. You can easily buy elderberry online or from any good health food retailer.

Natural Herpes Treatment Option: Herbs and Reishi Mushrooms

Certain herbs and spices are terrific (and easy) home remedies for herpes. Tribulus Terrestris, Astragalus, Cat's claw, galangal, lapacho and Cissus Quadrangularis are all anti-viral in nature and will help tremendously. Reishi mushrooms, ginger, turmeric, black pepper, cinnamon, cilantro (coriander), and the most powerful of them all, garlic, are also anti-viral and really give the immune system a strong boost. Cayenne pepper, licorice and thyme are three herbs that have actually been found to fight the herpes virus so be sure to use them in your cooking as much as possible (along with lots of garlic and cilantro). Remember, to successfully kill the herpes simplex virus you must detox your body, raise your pH level, and boost your immune system to the absolute maximum! This is crucial. All of these herbs and spices and mushrooms help to do this so it's vital you use them and consume them in high amounts every day.

Natural Herpes Cure: Natural Honey

Natural honey is an extremely powerful treatment for both HSV1 and HSV2. It's such a strong anti-viral and infection fighting food that it's still considered the number one remedy of choice by most natural therapists and alternative healers.

And a recent study has finally been able to validate the benefits of natural honey for treating herpe.

In the first part of the study, researchers treated 8 patients with genital herpes and 8 patients with oral herpes using Acyclovir as soon as a breakout occurred. In the second part of the study, they treated all 16 patients with honey instead of Acyclovir as soon as there was a second breakout and found that the healing time was 43% better for labial sores and 59% better for genital sores. Overall they found the length and extent of each attack, along with the duration of pain and healing time were much shorter with the honey than with Acyclovir. And with no side effects! Another study randomized 90 people with genital herpes and had them use one of three treatments during an outbreak... a propolis ointment (another bee/honey product), topical Zovirax, or a placebo ointment. They found the individuals in the propolis group experienced a much faster healing time for their lesions and were more likely to have fully healed sores by day 10 of the treatment compared to the people using Zovirax or the placebo.

How to Get the Most Out of the Honey Remedy

So, there are two ways to effectively use honey. Firstly, as an external remedy... When an outbreak occurs simply smear the honey (with a little coconut oil) on the affected area after urination and leave on for as long as possible. The second way is much easier... You simply eat it! Honey is not only anti-viral; it also contains nitric oxide metabolites. New research has indicated that increasing nitric oxide levels in bodily fluids may help retard and even prevent viral replication. This is of course welcome news for herpes sufferers. For best results, 1-2 tablespoons of honey should be eaten each day.

Manuka Honey is Best

Manuka honey is by far the most superior of all honeys. The pollen comes from the flowers of the potent medicinal plant known as the Manuka bush, found in Australia and New Zealand. Manuka honey has been proven to kill more than 250 bacterial strains and successfully treat the herpes simplex virus. This really is the only honey you should use. It's much stronger than natural honey, but with that said, if you only have access to natural honey or local honey then go ahead and use these. Natural honey is still a better option than using nothing at all. Whatever you do though, don't use processed honey (commercial honey sold in supermarkets) as this will actually make your symptoms much worse.

Apple cider vinegar is another terrific natural remedy and treatment for HSV1 and HSV2. It also contains some very potent anti-viral and infection-destroying properties and is actually one of the best detoxifiers and heavy metal removers in existence! As an added benefit, ACV helps to raise your bodies pH level and boost your immune system. Used topically, it also helps to relieve lesion pain and discomfort quite considerably. To get the most out of the ACV remedy, mix a tablespoon of organic apple cider vinegar containing the "mother" apple and a teaspoon of Manuka honey in a glass of warm filtered water and drink down. Do this 3 times a day on an empty stomach (first thing in the morning when you awake is especially important). If you find you can't handle the taste of the liquid ACV, go with the capsules instead. For external relief and to heal lesions faster, mix up a batch comprised of one cup ACV to one gallon of water. Soak with a wash cloth then use as a cold compress. Leave on the affected area for around 20 minutes. Repeat this process 2-3 times daily until all lesions are healed.

Hydrogen peroxide (HP): This should definitely be your first "go to" remedy when you have an outbreak. Hydrogen peroxide is also a very powerful internal parasitic cleanser and "oxygenator" (pH/alkaline booster). Because herpes is a parasite, and you also need to alkalize the body to destroy the virus, hydrogen peroxide is definitely a worthy (and cheap) addition to your daily treatment protocol. If you have a breakout, simply dilute some 12% grade hydrogen peroxide with clean filtered water (3 parts HP to 11 parts water for 3% solution) and apply directly to any lesions with a cotton ball. Do this 2-3 times a day and watch those sores disappear quicker than you've ever seen before. If you have a cold sore (HSV1), gently prick the sore with a sterilized needle then apply the HP with a cotton ball. Hold for at least 10 minutes. Be aware that the hydrogen peroxide may also bubble a bit in the beginning - this is normal. Make sure you use the 12% grade and dilute as directed above so it doesn't burn.Once you get down to the maintenance dose, however, rather than continue on this, drop the hydrogen peroxide completely then repeat the HP cycle/protocol again in another 3 months' time. After resting for 3 months, repeat the cycle once more before your 12 months is up.This seems to be the most effective method for using the hydrogen peroxide internally to destroy the virus. In addition to this, take a capful of 12% food grade hydrogen peroxide and mix with filtered or distilled water at a ratio of 3 parts HP to 11 parts water (becomes 3% solution) and gargle this every day after cleaning your teeth - do not swallow the mixture though, spit out afterwards. Bacteria and parasites live and breed in the mouth. Doing the HP gargle every day kills these unwanted pests, and in turn, enhances the assimilation and effectiveness of the food and supplements you'll be consuming quite significantly. Hydrogen peroxide also removes toxins and heavy metals from the body at a rapid rate via the above methods. Make sure you ONLY use food grade hydrogen peroxide for internal use and be sure to dilute accordingly. You can read more on all the in's and out's for using hydrogen peroxide to treat herpes in The One-Minute Cure book. Whatever you do though, do not pass up using this powerful cure!

NOTE: 35% food grade hydrogen peroxide (as per the books recommendation) is becoming increasingly difficult to obtain. This can be easily overcome, however, simply by purchasing the 12% solution and tripling the amount (12x3=36%) or purchasing the 8% solution and quadrupling the amount (8x4=32%) to give you your 35% grade.

DMSO: DMSO works a treat on all types of herpes outbreaks whether they be genital, cold sore or shingle related. As soon as you feel that tingling sensation coming on, apply a small amount of DMSO to the affected area. Do this 3 times a day for 3-4 days and either the outbreak won't happen at all, or it will be very mild and short lived. In addition to this, apply a small amount to the base of the spine, and if it's fever blisters (HSV1) that you have, also apply a small amount to the back of the neck (spine) and a tiny amount to the temples (trigeminal ganglia) where the virus resides when dormant. The great thing about DMSO is even if you have a full-blown breakout, it will still work. Buy the 70% DMSO solution in either liquid, cream or gel form. If you decide to go with the 99.9% pharmaceutical grade, make sure you water it down to a 70% solution before applying so it doesn't burn. In addition to this, you can mix the DMSO cream with the oregano oil (3-4 drops) and coconut oil when applying topically to the base of the spine (see #3 cure). DMSO helps penetrate the oregano oil deep into the ganglia nerve. Try and get the 70% DMSO cream with added aloe vera if you can as this helps to stop your skin drying out. HSV1 sufferers can also apply a small amount of the oregano oil/DMSO/coconut oil mix to the back of the neck and temples 3 times a week for extra benefit.

Tea tree oil: Tea tree oil is a virtual "cure all" topical treatment, and it works very well on herpes sores. Simply use a single drop from the eye dropper that comes with the bottle and rub lightly on the infected area.

Lemon balm: Lemon balm contains rosmarinic, caffeic and ferulic acid, the compounds which give this herb its potent anti-viral properties. It also works very well on skin lesions caused by the herpes virus. Buy the lemon balm liquid drops and apply 3-4 times a day.

Essential oils: Essential oils such as lavender and peppermint oil can also be used as a topical treatment.

However, we recommend you try these only if you don't receive any benefit from the lemon balm or tee tree oil as these are probably the least effective of the three for most people.

Aloe vera: This amazing plant will help with just about any ailment or skin condition you will ever encounter. It has no side effects and won't irritate or inflame the skin at all. Use the aloe vera creams or gels to provide some soothing relief to your herpes sores.

Myrrh: Myrrh contains potent anti-microbial, anti-bacterial, antiviral and antiseptic properties and is a powerful immune booster. The ancient Egyptians are said to have used this plant to cure herpes over 5000 years ago (yes, herpes was even around back then). You can use myrrh essential oil as a topical remedy for herpes lesions (and it works a treat for this), but where it really comes into its own is when it's taken internally. Myrrh extract resin doesn't just significantly enhance the body's immune response, it prompts the immune system to attack the virus whenever it tries to break out and go on a rampage at your expense. If you're going to use myrrh, make sure you follow the directions listed on the side of the bottle.

Some foods will definitely impair the healing process while others will help speed it up. The main "no no" is caffeine and any foods that contain it. Caffeine impairs the healing process like nothing else. Foods you must avoid include coffee, black tea and chocolate. However, we do strongly recommend you drink Matcha green tea every day for its potent health and healing benefits. Even though it contains a small amount of caffeine, Matcha green tea boosts the immune system and speeds up the healing process tremendously. In this case, the pros definitely outweigh any cons! The other foods and ingredients you need to avoid are all refined sugars and processed foods (including processed dairy), along with GMO's and hybrid foods. These man-altered disaster foods do absolutely nothing for your body and are laced with artificial additives and toxic chemicals that inhibit the effectiveness of the remedies we've just discussed. Tap water should also be avoided due to it's high heavy metal and pesticide content (and tap water can contain parasites and other unwanted pathogens) so make sure you only drink clean filtered water, and of course, no alcohol! You will most likely already feel tired and lethargic from the virus so why would you eat foods and drink liquids that are only going to make you more tired and lethargic anyway? Nuts (not seeds) are also on the list of foods to avoid as they seem to exacerbate the virus due to their high levels of arginine.

The foods you need to be eating more of are the basics... organic fruits (especially capers for quercetin flavonol, avocados and olives, along with apples and red grapes for resveratrol antioxidant), herbs and spices (especially LOTS of cilantro and turmeric), vegetables, fish (wild caught salmon, tuna and sardines), and omega 3 fatty acid seeds such as flax seeds, hemp and chia seeds. In addition, coconuts contain some very powerful anti-viral and infection fighting properties (specifically, a viral destroying substance called monolaurin), along with essential fatty acids, so make sure you consume plenty of organic coconut oil, coconut water, and take a high quality monolaurin supplement every day. Green foods such as wheat grass and the blue-green algae chlorella and spirulina are highly alkalizing and chelate (remove toxins and heavy metals) from the body. They are also high in organic iron (your immune system relies on iron to fight the virus) so try and add one or both of these to a morning smoothie every day, along with Atlantic dulse seaweed (another very powerful heavy metal remover) and the anti-viral fruits, pomegranate and maqui berries (you can buy these in powdered form). In addition, take a good quality probiotic supplement and eat plenty of cultured foods such as sauerkraut, kimchi and natural yogurt as well for a healthy gut and healthy digestion. Finally, make sure you eat LOTS of organic onions and garlic! Yes, this may seem a bit "out there" but many herpes sufferers are experiencing amazing results from drinking their own home-made onion and garlic broth. This makes sense as onions (particularly red onions) and garlic contain some of the most powerful anti-viral and immune boosting substances yet found, including the herpes destroying quercetin flavonol. And a 1992 study by Brigham Young University actually found that garlic was able to kill 90% of the herpes simplex virus within 30 minutes of applying it to a laboratory dish!s

www.ingramcontent.com/pod-product-compliance
Lightning Source LLC
Chambersburg PA
CBHW072142150726
48002CB00004B/1586